Vulnerable Populations and Medicare Services

Why Do Disparities Exist?

Marian E. Gornick

2000 • The Century Foundation Press • New York

The Century Foundation, formerly the Twentieth Century Fund, sponsors and supervises timely analyses of economic policy, foreign affairs, and domestic political issues. Not-for-profit and nonpartisan, it was founded in 1919 and endowed by Edward A. Filene.

Library of Congress Cataloging-in-Publication Data

Gornick, Marian.
Vulnerable populations and medicare services: why do disparities exist? / by Marian E. Gornick.
p. cm.
ISBN 0-87078-447-1
1. Medicare. 2. Medical care—Utilization—United States. 3. Medicare—Statistics. 4. Medical care—Utilization—United States—Statistics. I. Title.

RA412.3 .G67 2000
362.1'0973—dc21

99-089756

Cover design: Claude Goodwin
Manufactured in the United States of America.

Vulnerable Populations and Medicare Services

FOREWORD

The phrase "as long as you have your health" nicely conveys the fundamental importance of physical well-being throughout a person's life. For the poor, the uninsured, and the aged, the wording might be altered a bit to capture the reality of their situations, reading instead "as long as you can afford to pay for your health." This notion is particularly apt at the beginning of the twenty-first century, when technology and medicine have combined to make health itself seem—probably for the first time in human history—somewhat under our control. We talk of illness and health as though they were things that could be managed, given the necessary expertise and the proper treatments. Of course, for most people through their early and middle years, bad health is only a temporary inconvenience—a nasty cold or debilitating flu. But then, except for the lucky few who are both long-lived and healthy until the end, prescription drugs, doctor visits, and invasive tests become a routine part of life. In fact, many smart and talented people almost seem to take on a new career in retirement as managers of their personal health services.

These two concepts—the rise of health care consumption with age and the notion that a great many health problems can now be dealt with, given the right course of treatment—have combined in the past thirty years to make health-related issues increasingly important to more and more citizens. And so, as America ages, political leaders and voters have found themselves compelled to pay more attention to health matters. One engine driving this shift is the change in the share of expenditures on health, from 5 percent of gross domestic product less than a generation ago to 13.5 percent today. Since half of this money comes from the public sector (in effect, from taxes), the political importance of health issues is compelling.

Within the broad area of health concerns, two issues seem to loom largest—health care coverage for the uninsured and the future security of the Medicare program. The fact that Medicare exists at all seems something of a miracle in the current political environment. Medicare's passage in 1965 realized the promise made when Social Security was enacted three decades earlier—that no American need be destitute simply because he or she is too old to work. For those sixty-five or over, Medicare has made a huge difference (indeed, in some studies, it is associated with increases in longevity), but the program is not perfect. For one thing, with the probable large increase in the share of the population eligible for coverage during the next half century, the financial and political pressures on the program are expected by some observers to be severe. Nor does the program serve all populations equally well.

This report focuses on the disparities that persist under the Medicare program even after access to insurance coverage for the elderly has been equalized. Marian Gornick, who was with the Health Care Financing Administration (HCFA) for more than twenty years, has found evidence of this continuing problem in new data from HCFA. She explains that the available statistics before 1990 tended to mask disparities in care by race and socioeconomic status. Gornick argues that this story often has been overlooked in the emphasis on other, admittedly significant, health issues. She also offers policy recommendations for dealing with these disparities, starting with the need to call attention to them and to develop better systems for monitoring equity in health services as well as the importance of further research and analysis into this issue.

Gornick's findings of inequality are troubling and deserve attention. The Century Foundation is pleased to have supported this research and to present these important new data about inequalities in the utilization of Medicare.

RICHARD C. LEONE, *President*
The Century Foundation
January 2000

Contents

Acknowledgments

The author wishes to express appreciation for the support of The Century Foundation and the efforts of Greg Anrig, Leif Wellington Haase, Benjamin Aldrich-Moodie, and Sarah Nelson in overseeing the project and the preparation of the manuscript. I am also indebted to the helpful comments provided by two anonymous reviewers.

The author also wishes to thank The Commonwealth Fund, whose grant in a related project supported the development of information and knowledge about disparities in the use of Medicare services. The views presented here are those of the author and should not be attributed to The Commonwealth Fund, their staff, officers, or directors.

I am also sincerely grateful to my former colleagues on the staff of the Health Care Financing Administration—Paul Eggers, Renee Mentnech, Gerald Adler, and David Baugh—for sharing and developing current Medicare data to use in this project.

1

Introduction

In the years preceding the passage of the Social Security Act of 1935, minorities and the poor used less health care than others. Moreover, those aged sixty-five years and over had greater health care needs but less access to health insurance coverage than any other age group. These issues were lingering concerns until 1965, when Congress enacted health insurance for the aged.

The Medicare program filled a major gap in the nation's social welfare system. Virtually all of the elderly are entitled to hospital insurance (Part A) because eligibility is tied to Old-Age and Survivor's Insurance (OASI) under the Social Security system. Part B, the Supplementary Medical Insurance program, which covers physicians' and related services, is voluntary, but nearly all of the elderly participate through a premium paid by them or on their behalf.

Medicare's success in improving access to covered services was swift and dramatic. With the implementation of the program, the rate of charity care for hospital inpatients fell substantially for persons aged sixty-five and over. In Medicare's first year of operation, gaps in hospital admission rates and physician visits between elderly blacks and whites and between the rich and the poor declined.[1] Over time, the rate of hospital admissions for black beneficiaries reached—and then exceeded—the rate for white beneficiaries. These successes led to the conclusion that the

Medicare program was well on its way toward achieving its goal of providing equal access to care for all of the elderly.

Recognition of Disparities in Access

Until this decade, Medicare data were not detailed enough to caution us that hospital discharge rates were not precise enough an indicator of access to services.[2] Nearly a quarter of a century elapsed from the time Medicare became operational (1966) until the time when Medicare data were sufficiently detailed (1990) to recognize that even though hospital discharge rates were equalized, the rate of use of specific Medicare services was associated with race and socioeconomic status.[3] Detailed data became available when Congress mandated changes in the methods used by Medicare to pay hospitals and physicians. The new payment formulas required information on the patient's diagnoses and the specific medical and surgical services utilized. This information provided a much more detailed data set than previously available. It revealed that there were substantial disparities in the use of specific Medicare-covered services, including nearly every common surgery elderly patients undergo in the hospital, such as coronary artery bypass surgery and hip and knee replacement.

The major purpose of this report is to inform policymakers and health care experts about the kinds of disparities in Medicare utilization that are obvious now—and to awaken concern and interest in taking steps toward equalizing access to care.

Defining Access

Access to care has two dimensions: "potential access," which refers to resources that affect whether individuals can enter into the health care system, such as health insurance coverage, and "realized access," which refers to their actual entry into the health care system[4]—for example, use of physicians' visits. In this report, realized access is analyzed first by comparing Medicare utilization rates for a number of services across subgroups of the elderly. Then, potential access is examined by considering which factors may be associated with vulnerable subgroups of the Medicare-covered population that may influence disparities in Medicare utilization.

To evaluate whether differences in utilization rates across population subgroups are a cause for concern, it is necessary to consider the need for services, and groups can differ in need. For example, elderly whites have higher rates of osteoporosis and thus can be expected to be hospitalized for hip fracture repair more frequently than blacks. In contrast, elderly blacks have higher rates of diabetes, hypertension, and other chronic conditions and thus can be expected to need more physicians' services for effective management of these conditions than whites.

To put Medicare utilization patterns into perspective, this report first discusses important measures of health, such as mortality and morbidity, for various subgroups of the elderly. Then Medicare utilization patterns for these subgroups are analyzed.[5] This approach allows us to identify subgroups of the elderly vulnerable to poor health and to compare their use of Medicare services with the use of services by less vulnerable subgroups. This report was stimulated by the recognition that the use of many Medicare services by subgroups of the elderly is often in contrast to what these subgroups are expected to need.

Present Concerns

A further stimulus for this report was the finding that disparities in life expectancy between blacks and whites and between the rich and the poor are growing. Changes in health care delivery could widen this gap in life expectancy at an accelerated pace. Expansion of enrollment in managed care could have the unintended effect of exacerbating disparities in health care, if disadvantaged groups are less able to adapt to the intricacies of the new delivery systems.[6]

Various professional journals have published studies about the association of race and socioeconomic status with the use of Medicare services, but these studies have not made an impact significant enough to effect a change. Perhaps this is because these studies tend to single out a particular set of procedures—such as coronary artery procedures—or because the studies offer little in the way of explanations for disparities in Medicare utilization. To address these limitations, this report highlights disparities in the use of many different types of services and identifies potential causes and explanations. Although relatively few studies are available to draw upon in order to determine which factors are most influential in causing disparities in Medicare utilization, I hope that policy experts and the health care community can use the information presented here to take some needed steps toward ameliorating the significant disparities in Medicare utilization.

The unanticipated differences in the use of Medicare services across vulnerable subgroups of the elderly demonstrate that the implementation of a health insurance program does not, in and of itself, assure equal access to health care. Still, disparities in Medicare and other programs will not be eliminated by abandoning the hopes and goals of health care programs, in effect "throwing out the baby with the bath water." Health policy experts should weigh the potential causes and explanations for disparities in Medicare utilization and consider what steps can be taken toward achieving program goals of improving access to health care.

The ideas in this report are developed along five lines of inquiry, each explored in a chapter framed around a specific question.

- Chapter 2 addresses the question: What were Medicare's original goals, and what did early assessments reveal? It discusses the issues that stimulated the enactment of Medicare and the goals and expectations of the program. Summarizing findings from early assessments of the program (1967–90), it shows that global measures of utilization are insufficient to monitor health care use.

- Chapter 3 discusses: What disparities exist in the health of the elderly? It presents several measures of health status across vulnerable subgroups of the elderly, including trends in life expectancy at age sixty-five from 1969 to 1995. A number of morbidity and disability measures are also discussed.

- Chapter 4 addresses: What disparities exist in the use of Medicare services? It identifies specific patterns of Medicare utilization by race and socioeconomic status and juxtaposes these patterns with what was learned about disparities in health in Chapter 3. It shows that patterns of Medicare utilization by vulnerable subgroups of the elderly are not consistent with health care needs.

- Chapter 5 deals with the question: What are probable explanations for disparities in use? It examines several potential explanations for disparities in Medicare utilization and discusses which of these explanations are the most probable.

- Chapter 6 concludes by addressing: What steps can be taken toward bringing about a change? It makes recommendations that focus on three major issues: the wide dissemination of information about patterns in Medicare use, the creation of new data systems capable of monitoring access and equity in health care, and the development of a major research and experimentation agenda.

2

What Were Medicare's Original Goals, and What Did Early Assessments Reveal?

Medicare's primary goal of improving access to care for all of the elderly was stimulated by a landmark event that took place in 1927, when several philanthropic organizations sponsored a commission—known as the Committee on the Costs of Medical Care (CCMC)—to study the costs of medical services, their distribution, and how to pay for them. Their study, covering the period from 1928 to 1931, showed that rich families used more health care services than other families, while middle income families used health care at a rate closer to the rate for poor families than for rich families.[1] Although the CCMC did not recommend compulsory government health insurance, they recommended far-reaching changes in the organization and financing of medicine, including group payment for health care through taxation or private health insurance.

Another influence was Franklin Delano Roosevelt's 1944 State of the Union Message, which addressed the issue of medical care. Although FDR did not recommend government health insurance in this message, he advocated an "Economic Bill of Rights" that included "the right to adequate medical care and the opportunity to achieve and enjoy good health."[2]

By 1950, according to Paul Starr, a shift in the distribution of health care had occurred: medical care utilization by middle-income families approached the rate of rich families and "the poor stood out as different." He describes this shift as "a change from mass exclusion to minority exclusion from medical care."[3]

As public policy interest in access to medical care intensified, the group aged sixty-five and over were a particular concern. A high proportion of this age group lived at or below the poverty level, and most were no longer in the labor force, which meant that employer-sponsored health insurance was generally unavailable to them. Older persons had the option of purchasing individual health insurance, but individual policies were costly. Estimates show that about 50 percent of the elderly had hospital insurance, but minority and low-income persons were much less likely to be insured. These concerns influenced the development of the programs in the early 1960s, which "aimed specifically at reducing the exclusion from medical care of the poor and the aged."[4] After decades of debate, the Medicare and Medicaid programs were enacted into law on July 30, 1965, to provide access to care for the most vulnerable persons in the nation.

Early Assessment of the Impact of Medicare on Access: 1967–1990

As noted earlier, Medicare data files have been maintained centrally to administer the program (thus referred to as Medicare administrative data) and for program evaluation.[5] Ongoing monitoring of Medicare utilization depends upon the administrative data. Enrollment files are used for such information as the beneficiary's age, sex, and race. The claims files are used for information about the services paid for under the Medicare program.

During the first two decades of the Medicare program, information in the claims files was sufficient to analyze hospital discharge rates or physician visit rates—by age, sex, and race—but the administrative data could not be used to analyze rates of use of a specific procedure, such as coronary artery bypass graft, because this data set did not maintain specific procedure codes.

This limitation in the administrative data permitted only broad analyses of the use of services by age, sex, and race such as comparisons of hospital discharge rates, the proportion of beneficiaries who saw a physician at least once a year, or the number of visits per year. Surveys were used to analyze questions that required socioeconomic and health information. During the first two decades of the Medicare program several studies evaluated the impact of Medicare on access to services. It is instructive to review the types of analyses made in three of these studies—and to understand why their findings suggested that disparities by race and income had largely disappeared.

One study used survey data to compare utilization in the year preceding Medicare (1965) and during the first full year of the program (1967).[6] In 1965, the hospital discharge rate for the most affluent persons was 30 percent higher than for the least affluent, but this difference disappeared by 1967. The study also showed that 17 percent of all hospital stays for the elderly in 1965 were charity cases, whereas in 1967 this was reduced to 3 percent. The proportion of charges paid directly by the patient fell from 38 percent in 1965 to 7 percent in 1967.

A second study also used survey data to analyze insurance coverage and the use of health care services in the pre-Medicare period, 1963 to 1965, and during the eleven years after Medicare began.[7] For the earlier period, the study found that (1) more than 70 percent of the middle- and highest-income groups had health insurance, but only 44 percent of the group with the lowest income were insured; (2) the lowest-income group used less physician care than others; and (3) nonwhite elderly persons were admitted for hospital services at about half the rate for elderly whites. But in 1977, eleven years after Medicare began, although elderly whites were more likely to see a physician, of all patients who saw a physician, nonwhites had more visits. Although hospital use was still lower for nonwhites compared to whites, the gap was closing.

A third study used Medicare administrative data and analyzed the use of services for the first ten years of the program, from 1967 to 1976.[8] In 1967, the ratio of the number of minority persons who used inpatient care per 1,000 minority enrollees to the corresponding number of white persons was only 0.73, but by 1976 this ratio increased to 0.84. Similarly, the ratio of the number of minority persons who used physician services to the number of white persons who used physician services rose from 0.67 in 1967 to 0.86 in 1976.[9]

Although available data were limited, these three studies illustrated that access to services vastly increased after Medicare was implemented. Moreover, the fact that Medicare beneficiaries no longer had to rely on charity care indicated to most analysts that the major barriers to health care were eliminated.

It is significant to note, however, that two public health experts reviewed the available Medicare studies and each recommended caution in interpreting the results. Avedis Donabedian noted that although Medicare and Medicaid studies suggested that access to hospital and physicians' services improved for lower-income persons in the United States, available data were not sufficient to reliably evaluate the impacts of these programs.[10] He observed that "perhaps a reasonable conclusion is that the use of services nationwide is still not congruent with need."

Karen Davis reviewed the literature in 1991 and acknowledged the improvement shown in access to care in the Medicare studies.[11] Nonetheless, she observed that studies more recent than these illustrated the importance of a growing trend toward using disaggregated data to "look at specific services and the link between access to health services and health outcomes." Davis cited a study that found that black women had a higher incidence of invasive cervical cancer but a lower rate of pap smears, concluding that there was a need for better data and programs targeted to high-risk populations.

Later Assessment of the Impact of Medicare on Access

Medicare data showed that over time hospital discharge rates among the elderly continued to increase faster for blacks than for whites. By 1986, the ratio of the hospital discharge rate for blacks to the rate for whites reached 1.03; by 1992 it was 1.10.[12]

Disaggregated data are available now that permit us to analyze not just hospital discharge rates but also the use of specific Medicare services across subgroups of the elderly. As background information on the health of various subgroups of the elderly, Chapter 3 provides different health status measures for these subgroups. Then Chapter 4 provides information on disparities in the use of specific Medicare services.

3

What Disparities Exist in the Health of the Elderly?

In the United States and many other industrialized nations, health is strongly associated with socioeconomic status.[1] The concept of socioeconomic status provides a framework for understanding how certain social and economic characteristics of individuals (typically income, education, and occupation) relate to their place in society. Some of the causal links between socioeconomic status and health are self-evident: families at the higher end of the income and education scales have more resources than others to choose nutritious diets, healthy behaviors, safe neighborhoods, and safe occupations. Clearly, Medicare could not have been expected to affect all of the aspects of society associated with health. However, it was expected to weaken the links between socioeconomic status and health care. This, in turn, was expected to ameliorate disparities in health (alternatively described as health status or health outcomes).

In the United States, there is also a strong association between health and race—although the influence of race and socioeconomic status is often intertwined and difficult to disentangle. In all age groups, the health status of black Americans is lower, on average, than that of white Americans. Differences in rates of illness between blacks and whites for certain health conditions are consistent with known differences in biological or genetic makeup; a well-known example is the higher rate of sickle cell anemia among American blacks. In general, however, there are no known biological or genetic explanations for the higher rates of illness and disabling conditions in blacks compared to whites. Rather, differences in health are believed to reflect the effects of socioeconomic and minority status.

Health status in the United States is also associated with membership in racial and ethnic minority groups other than blacks and whites; however, these relationships are not always consistent. For example, in 1996, death rates for Hispanic males fifteen to forty-four years of age were higher than the rates for non-Hispanic white males in that age group, but for all ages combined, mortality rates for Hispanic males were about 20 percent lower than for non-Hispanic white males.[2] The relatively low death rate found for older Hispanics, including those of Mexican origin, is remarkable because of their relatively low income and educational levels. Also remarkable is the fact that death rates for persons in the United States of Asian/Pacific Island origin are the lowest of the four racial categories that the federal government has established for statistical reporting.[3] The comparatively low death rates for older Hispanics and Asian/Pacific Islanders are believed to reflect to some extent selective immigration and cultural attributes that continue among these groups in the United States and that influence positive health outcomes.[4]

Mortality is but one useful indicator of health.[5] The association between health and socioeconomic (or minority) status is generally consistent over time and over different measures of health—including mortality, morbidity, and disability.[6] However, the relationships can change over time; as ethnic groups undergo acculturation, the protective factors associated with their country of origin can decline. An example often cited is the increase in the rate of heart disease among those of Japanese origin who live in Hawaii. Another example is the rise in hypertension among those of Mexican origin who have settled in the United States.[7]

Studies in the United States tend to highlight the association between health and race/ethnicity rather than exploring the links between health and socioeconomic status.[8] The continuing concerns about the health of racial- and ethnic-minority groups in the United States has influenced the type of data we collect. Information is collected more often on race/ethnicity than on income, education, and occupation. Because minority groups in the United States generally have lower incomes and educational attainment, and are more frequently employed in lower-status occupations, many studies use race/ethnicity as a proxy for socioeconomic status.[9] When disparities are found in health across racial and ethnic minority groups, they are often assumed to reflect primarily their lower socioeconomic status. Although that is a generally valid assumption, studies that have been able to control for socioeconomic status often find that disparities in health status between blacks and whites do not entirely disappear.

Disparities in Socioeconomic Status and in Health

Income and Education

The assumption that there are substantial disparities in income and education by race and ethnicity is readily supported by the Medicare Current Beneficiary Survey (MCBS). As shown in Table 3.1 (page 16), in 1996 the percentage of elderly whites with incomes over $25,000 (33 percent) was far greater than the percentage of blacks (10 percent) or Hispanics (11 percent). The percentage of whites who completed high school was also greater than the percentage of blacks or Hispanics. As expected, income and education are highly correlated: among whites, blacks, and Hispanics in the higher income groups, a greater proportion had a high school education than in the lower income group.

TABLE 3.1
INCOME AND EDUCATIONAL STATUS OF WHITE, BLACK, AND HISPANIC MEDICARE BENEFICIARIES AGE SIXTY-FIVE AND OVER, 1996

	ALL INCOMES	INCOME ≤ $25,000	INCOME ≥ $25,001
Total number of beneficiaries	35.5 million	25.1 million	10.4 million
White	29.4 million (100%)	19.7 million (67%)	9.7 million (33%)
Black	3.1 million (100%)	2.8 million (90%)	0.3 million (10%)
Hispanic	2.2 million (100%)	2.0 million (89%)	0.2 million (11%)
Completed high school (percent)			
White	65	55	86
Black	37	33	79
Hispanic	30	25	75

Source: Medicare Current Beneficiary Survey, 1996; unpublished tabulations provided by the Health Care Financing Administration.

DISPARITIES IN HEALTH AMONG ELDERLY SUBGROUPS

Life expectancy at age sixty-five (remaining years of life). In the early years of the Medicare program (1969–71), the gap in life expectancy in the United States between black men and white men at age sixty-five was only 0.5 years, and the gap between black women and white women was 1.2 years (see Table 3.2). Over the next quarter century, the gap widened. By 1995, at age sixty-five, white men and white women could expect to live two full years longer than their black counterparts. Life expectancy during the twenty-five-year period, while increasing for men and women of both races, increased 2.7 years for elderly white males but only 1.1 years for elderly black males. Similarly, life expectancy at age sixty-five for elderly white

TABLE 3.2
LIFE EXPECTANCY IN THE UNITED STATES AT AGE SIXTY-FIVE IN YEARS, BY RACE AND SEX, SELECTED TIME PERIODS

	1969–71	1979–81	1994	1995
Males				
White	13.0	14.3	15.6	15.7
Black	12.5	13.3	13.6	13.6
Gap (years)	0.5	1.0	2.0	2.1
Females				
White	16.9	18.6	19.1	19.1
Black	15.7	17.1	17.2	17.1
Gap (years)	1.2	1.5	1.9	2.0

Sources: "Vital Statistics of the United States, 1994," preprint of vol. II, Mortality, part A, sec. 6 life tables (Hyattsville, Md.: National Center for Health Statistics, 1998); and R. N. Anderson, K. D. Kochanek, and S. L. Murphy, "Report of Final Mortality Statistics, 1995," *Monthly Vital Statistics Report* 45, no. 11, supp. 2 (Hyattsville, Md.: National Center for Health Statistics, 1997), Table 4.

females increased by 2.2 years, compared to only 1.4 years for black females.

The effects of income on mortality rates. In addition to race, income is associated with mortality rates among the elderly enrolled in Medicare. As shown in Table 3.3 (page 18), the number of deaths per 100 beneficiaries aged sixty-five years and over in 1993 was higher for black males (8.0 deaths) than for white males (6.7 deaths); similarly, the mortality rate was higher for black women (5.2 deaths) than for white women (4.5 deaths). Among men of both races, the death rate declined as income increased. This was most notable for white men, with the number falling from 7.3 deaths per 100 white men with incomes less than or equal to $13,000 to 6.2 deaths per 100 white men with incomes equal to or greater than $20,501. For women of both races, the death rate was fairly flat across income groups.

TABLE 3.3
NUMBER OF DEATHS PER 100 MEDICARE BENEFICIARIES AGE SIXTY-FIVE AND OVER PER YEAR, BY RACE, SEX, AND INCOME, 1993

		Income			
	Mean	≤ $13,000	$13,101– $16,300	$16,301– $20,500	≥ $20,501
Males					
Black	8.0	8.1	8.0	7.8	7.7
White	6.7	7.3	7.1	6.8	6.2
Females					
Black	5.2	5.2	5.3	5.0	5.3
White	4.5	4.6	4.5	4.5	4.4

Source: *Monitoring the Impact of Medicare Physician Payment Reform on Utilization and Access; 1995 Report to Congress,* HCFA pub. no. 03379 (Baltimore, Md.: Health Care Financing Administration, 1995).

Leading causes of death. Mortality rates among persons in the United States aged sixty-five and over differ substantially by race and ethnicity (see Table 3.4). For all causes combined, the death rate per 100,000 persons aged sixty-five and over in 1995 was 5,679 for blacks, 5,049 for whites, and 3,178 for Hispanics. For the three leading causes of death among the aged (heart disease, cancer, and stroke), the rate for blacks exceeded the rate for whites and Hispanics. Death rates for blacks were also higher than whites and Hispanics for diabetes mellitus; accidents and adverse events; nephritis, nephrotic syndrome, and nephrosis; septicemia; and hypertension. In brief, elderly blacks are at a greater risk of death than whites or Hispanics from the majority of major conditions that threaten the life of the elderly.

Cancer: death rates, stage, and five-year survival. As already noted, the death rate from cancer is substantially higher for elderly blacks than elderly whites. As shown in Table 3.5 (page 20),

TABLE 3.4
TEN LEADING CAUSES OF DEATH AND RATE PER 100,000 FOR PERSONS AGE SIXTY-FIVE AND OVER, BY RACE AND ETHNICITY, UNITED STATES 1995

Cause of death	Total Rate	White Rate	Black Rate	Hispanic Rate
All causes	5,053	5,049	5,679	3,178
Diseases of the heart	1,835	1,842	2,006	1,118
Malignant neoplasms	1,137	1,129	1,348	681
Cerebrovascular diseases	414	410	493	242
Chronic obstructive pulmonary disease	264	276	169	126
Pneumonia and influenza	222	224	206	138
Diabetes mellitus	133	123	247	191
Accidents and adverse events	87	87	91	61
Alzheimer	60	63	—	—
Nephritis, nephrotic syndrome, and nephrosis	60	56	109	37
Septicemia	50	—	95	28
Atherosclerosis	—	49	—	—
Hypertension	—	—	72	—
Chronic liver disease and cirrhosis	—	—	—	54

Source: R. N. Anderson, K. D. Kochanek, and S. L. Murphy, "Report of Final Mortality Statistics, 1995," *Monthly Vital Statistics Report* 45, no. 11, supp. 2 (Hyattsville, Md.: National Center for Health Statistics, 1997), Tables 7 and 15.

except for breast and bladder cancer, mortality rates for each of the major cancer sites shown are higher for elderly blacks than for elderly whites. For prostate cancer the death rate per 100,000 black men (476 deaths) was more than twice the death rate for white men (220 deaths).

The higher death rates generally found for elderly black patients with cancer very likely reflect the fact that fewer black patients have localized cancer when first diagnosed. Data from the

TABLE 3.5

MORTALITY RATES FOR ALL CANCERS AND FOR SPECIFIC SITES FOR PERSONS AGE SIXTY-FIVE AND OVER, BY RACE AND SEX, 1988–92 (AVERAGE ANNUAL DEATHS PER 100,000)

	White Rate			Black Rate		
Site of Cancer	Total	Male	Female	Total	Male	Female
All Sites	1060	1441	822	1314	1982	912
Colon and rectum	132	167	110	157	191	137
Lung and bronchus	296	468	181	328	599	159
Urinary bladder	26	48	14	26	38	18
Breast	78	1.5	128	78	2.7	125
Corpus and uterus (females)	22	—	22	40	—	40
Prostate (males)	220	220	—	476	476	—

Source: C. L. Kosary et al., eds., "SEER Cancer Statistics Review, 1973–1992: Tables and Graphs," NIH pub. no. 96-2789 (Bethesda, Md.: National Cancer Institute, 1995).

Surveillance, Epidemiology, and End Results (SEER) cancer registries indicate that for each of the major cancer sites in Table 3.5, black patients are less likely to have localized cancer when they are first diagnosed. Among patients with prostate cancer, 52 percent of black men had localized cancer at the time of diagnosis compared to 58 percent of white men (see Table 3.6). The disparities in the rate of localized cancer are notable for the two cancers sites that primarily affect women—breast cancer and cancer of the corpus and uterus; among black women the percentage with localized cancer at the time of diagnosis was 48 percent for breast cancer and 52 percent for cancer of the corpus and uterus, while the corresponding figures for white women were 59 percent and 74 percent, respectively.

For each of the major cancer sites, there are notable disparities by race in five-year survival rates for patients diagnosed between the ages of sixty-five and seventy-four. As shown in Table 3.6, among men diagnosed with prostate cancer at ages sixty-five to seventy-four, 76.0 percent of black men survived five years compared to 90.9 percent of white men. Among women diagnosed with breast cancer at ages sixty-five to seventy-four, only 73.1 percent of black women survived compared to 86.7 percent of white women. Corresponding survival rates for cancer of the corpus and uterus were 45.2 percent for black women and 84.8 percent for white women.

Morbidity and disability. Rates of disease and disability, as well as other indicators, such as self-reported health status, provide information about the health of elderly subgroups that mortality alone does not disclose, especially when income is considered. In 1996, for example, among elderly Medicare beneficiaries of all

TABLE 3.6
PERCENT OF PATIENTS WITH LOCALIZED CANCER AT TIME OF DIAGNOSIS, AND PERCENT OF PATIENTS SURVIVING FIVE YEARS, BY RACE, 1986–91

	WHITE		BLACK	
Site of cancer	Percent with localized cancer when diagnosed[a]	Percent surviving five years[b]	Percent with localized cancer when diagnosed[a]	Percent surviving five years[b]
All Sites	—	57.0	—	42.5
Colon and rectum	38	64.0	32	51.4
Lung and bronchus	15	13.5	13	9.9
Urinary bladder	74	82.5	58	59.3
Breast	59	86.7	48	73.1
Corpus and uterus	74	84.8	52	45.2
Prostate	58	90.9	52	76.0

[a] all ages
[b] ages 65–74

Source: C. L. Kosary et al., eds., "SEER Cancer Statistics Review, 1973–1992: Tables and Graphs," NIH pub. no. 96-2789 (Bethesda, Md.: National Cancer Institute, 1995).

incomes combined, 44 percent of Hispanics, 42 percent of blacks, and 25 percent of whites reported their health as only fair or poor. However, among those with incomes over $25,000, only 21 percent of Hispanics, 29 percent of blacks, and 16 percent of whites rated their health as fair or poor. By contrast, among those with incomes of $25,000 or less, 46 percent of Hispanics, 43 percent of blacks, and 29 percent of whites reported this. (See Table 3.7.)

The presence of certain chronic conditions is frequently related to race and ethnicity. For all incomes combined, diabetes was reported by 25 percent of all elderly blacks and Hispanics, compared to only 13 percent of whites. Similarly, hypertension was more frequently reported by elderly blacks and Hispanics compared to whites.

Race and ethnicity as well as income are all associated with reported limitations in activities of daily living (ADL) and in

TABLE 3.7

PERCENT OF MEDICARE BENEFICIARIES AGE SIXTY-FIVE AND OVER REPORTING SELECTED HEALTH STATUS MEASURES, BY RACE AND HISPANIC ORIGIN AND BY INCOME, 1996

	Percent		
	White	Black	Hispanic
Rates health fair or poor			
All incomes	25	42	44
$25,000 or lower	29	43	46
$25,001 or higher	16	29	21
Has diabetes			
All incomes	13	25	25
$25,000 or lower	15	24	25
$25,001 or higher	12	27	18
Has hypertension			
All incomes	49	67	55
$25,000 or lower	51	66	56
$25,001 or higher	45	70	46

Source: Medicare Current Beneficiary Survey for 1996; unpublished data provided by the Health Care Financing Administration.

instrumental activities of daily living (IADL). The proportion of elderly blacks who reported having functional limitations (53 percent) was higher than elderly whites (43 percent) and Hispanics (49 percent). The effect of income on limitations in ADL and IADL is striking; among blacks, whites, and Hispanics, the proportion reporting such functional limitations was about 50 percent among those with incomes of $25,000 or less, compared to only about 30 percent in the higher income group. (See Table 3.8.)

TABLE 3.8
PERCENT OF MEDICARE BENEFICIARIES AGE SIXTY-FIVE AND OVER REPORTING LIMITATIONS IN IADL OR ADL, BY RACE AND HISPANIC ORIGIN AND BY INCOME, 1996

	Percent		
	White	Black	Hispanic
All incomes	43	53	49
$25,000 or lower	50	55	51
$25,001 or higher	29	33	29

Source: Medicare Current Beneficiary Survey for 1996; unpublished data provided by the Health Care Financing Administration.

SUMMARY

Since the early days of the Medicare program, life expectancy for white men and women at age sixty-five has increased more rapidly than for their black counterparts. Elderly Hispanics have lower mortality rates than whites, but they report more illness and disability than whites, particularly diabetes, hypertension, and limitations in ADL and IADL.

Socioeconomic status is clearly associated with health status. This is especially noticeable among white men aged sixty-five and over, whose mortality rates increase steadily as income declines. Low income elderly are more likely to report that their health is only fair or poor and that they have functional limitations, compared to more advantaged elderly.

Cancer mortality for elderly blacks is higher for nearly every major site compared to elderly whites. In addition, the percent of patients with localized cancer at the time of diagnosis is much lower for blacks than for whites, indicating that blacks, when first diagnosed, are more likely to have cancer that has advanced to a more invasive stage. This fact very likely contributes to their higher rates of death due to cancer.

4

What Disparities Exist in the Use of Medicare Services?

The information in this chapter was drawn from Medicare administrative data. Beginning in the mid-1980s, this data system began to maintain information newly available in the claims on the use of specific services that Medicare beneficiaries received in the fee-for-service sector. Data for 1996 represent about 88 percent of all elderly beneficiaries. The remaining 12 percent were enrolled in managed care systems.

Utilization patterns can be drawn reliably only for white and black enrollees, although an effort is under way to update race and ethnicity codes. To analyze the effects of socioeconomic status on the use of Medicare services, Medicare enrollment files were linked to data on median income at the ZIP code level derived from the 1990 U.S. census.

Disparities in the use of Medicare services became evident for the first time when utilization rates for fourteen common surgeries were analyzed for patients hospitalized in 1986.[1] Unexpectedly, the rate for each of these fourteen procedures was found to be greater for white beneficiaries than for black beneficiaries, and the differences (for example, for coronary artery bypass surgery) were often substantial. This led to the development of a system to classify all Medicare-covered Part B services into a manageable number of categories and to monitor utilization on an ongoing basis.[2] Although Medicare covers hundreds of services, a relatively small number of services were selected for this chapter to illustrate patterns of utilization across subgroups of the elderly.

As the next set of tables show, utilization patterns—viewed in light of what is known about the health of vulnerable subgroups of the elderly—raise a number of concerns.

Disparities in the Use of Medicare Services

Physicians' Visits

In 1996, the black to white ratio of physician office visits was 0.82, indicating that black beneficiaries received 18 percent fewer office visits than whites. However, blacks received more visits than whites while in the hospital and in the emergency room (see Table 4.1). In light of the findings from Chapter 3 that elderly blacks have poorer health—and thus would need continuous and comprehensive care from physicians at least as frequently as elderly whites—these patterns of Medicare utilization suggest that ongoing medical care and management of health are less accessible to black beneficiaries than to white beneficiaries.

Moreover, elderly blacks had 23 percent fewer specialist visits than elderly whites. In particular, blacks had 11 percent fewer visits from ophthalmologists, even though eye disease, especially glaucoma, is more prevalent among blacks than whites.[3]

Influenza Immunizations

In 1993, Medicare began to cover influenza immunization, a service recommended for all of the elderly. Because influenza is often a forerunner to pneumonia and is responsible for excess Medicare hospitalizations among the elderly with heart and pulmonary disease, flu immunization is considered one of Medicare's most important preventive services.[4]

In the fee-for-service sector in 1993, only 17.3 percent of elderly blacks were immunized, compared to 36.5 percent of whites (see Table 4.2, page 28). Although there has been an increase over time in the rate of flu immunizations for both races, in 1997 only about one in four elderly blacks received flu immunizations paid for by Medicare, as opposed to nearly one in two whites. (Any flu shots provided without charge to the Medicare program are not included in these rates.) Socioeconomic status is also related to the use of influenza immunization. In 1993, the immunization rate among the least-affluent white beneficiaries was 26 percent lower than among the most affluent whites, and

Table 4.1
Physician Visit Rates for Medicare Enrollees Age Sixty-five and Over, by Race, 1996

Type of Visit	White (rate per 100)	Black (rate per 100)	Ratio (black:white)
Office	604	498	0.82
Hospital: Inpatient	287	396	1.38
Emergency Room	39	55	1.40
Home/Nursing home	70	89	1.28
Specialists: All types	207	160	0.77
Ophthalmology[a]	84	75	0.89
Consultations	74	82	1.10
Chiropractic	46	8.5	0.19

[a]Ophthalmology visits included in Specialists: All types.

Source: Part B Monitoring System (age-adjusted rates), data supplied by Paul Eggers, Health Care Financing Administration.

among the least-affluent black beneficiaries the rate was 39 percent lower than among the most affluent.[5] These differences by race and socioeconomic status cannot be attributed to financial barriers (flu shots require no cost-sharing), but rather they indicate that there are other barriers that blacks and disadvantaged beneficiaries experience more frequently than whites and advantaged beneficiaries.

TABLE 4.2
INFLUENZA IMMUNIZATION RATES FOR MEDICARE ENROLLEES AGE SIXTY-FIVE AND OVER, BY RACE, 1993–1997

	White (rate per 100)	Black (rate per 100)	Ratio (black:white)
1993	36.5	17.3	0.47
1994	41.9	20.6	0.49
1995	43.2	21.6	0.50
1996	45.5	23.4	0.51
1997	46.1	24.3	0.53

Source: Health Care Financing Administration, Office of Information Services, National Claims History and Denominator File. Data developed by the Office of Strategic Planning and Office of Clinical Standards and Quality.

MAMMOGRAPHY

Mammography screening became a covered benefit under Medicare on January 1, 1991. Mammograms were heralded as an important new service because mammography rates among older women—who face a greater risk of developing breast cancer than younger women—were consistently lower than for younger women. During the period from 1992 to 1993, only 28.1 percent of black women received mammograms compared to 38.2 percent of white women, indicating that black women received 26 percent fewer mammograms than white women (see Table 4.3). Over time, the rates increased for women of both races, but in

1996–97 the rate for black women was still 21 percent lower than for white women. Similar to influenza immunization patterns, mammography rates are lower for the least affluent women of both races.

In view of the fact that black women are more likely to have later-stage breast cancer when first diagnosed and have lower five-year survival rates after diagnosis, there is a pressing need to understand the reasons for the disparities in the use of mammography services by elderly women.

Diagnostic Services

Sigmoidoscopy and colonoscopy are commonly performed for diagnosing colon abnormalities. In 1996, sigmoidoscopy rates were 39 percent lower and colonoscopy rates were 12 percent lower for black beneficiaries than for white beneficiaries (see Table 4.4, page 30). These disparities—in light of the fact that blacks have a higher rate of late-stage colon cancer and a higher death rate due to colon cancer—raise concerns about whether there are differences by race in access to quality medical care for patients at risk of colon cancer.

Similar concerns are raised by the disparities in the use of sonography of the carotid artery. This procedure is used for

Table 4.3
Mammography Rates for Medicare Enrollees Age Sixty-five and Over, by Race, 1992–1997

	White women (rate per 100)	Black women (rate per 100)	Ratio (black:white)
1992–93	38.2	28.1	0.74
1994–95	40.4	30.9	0.77
1996–97	42.5	33.7	0.79

Source: Health Care Financing Administration, Office of Information Services, National Claims History and Denominator File. Data developed by the Office of Strategic Planning and Office of Clinical Standards and Quality.

diagnosing occlusion of the carotid artery, a condition that can lead to stroke. As shown in Table 4.4, sonography of the carotid artery was performed at a 24 percent lower rate for elderly blacks compared to elderly whites.

TABLE 4.4
RATES OF SELECTED ENDOSCOPY AND SONOGRAPHY PROCEDURES FOR MEDICARE ENROLLEES AGE SIXTY-FIVE AND OVER, BY RACE, 1996

	White (rate per 1,000)	Black (rate per 1,000)	Ratio (black:white)
Endoscopy			
Sigmoidoscopy	34	21	0.61
Colonoscopy	56	49	0.88
Sonography			
Carotid Artery	65	49	0.76

Source: Part B Monitoring System (age-adjusted rates), data supplied by Paul Eggers, Health Care Financing Administration.

ELECTIVE PROCEDURES

As noted earlier, data for Medicare patients hospitalized in 1986 revealed that the use of common elective procedures was substantially less frequent for black beneficiaries than for white beneficiaries. In 1996, as Table 4.5 shows, differences by race in the use of common elective procedures continue. Two procedures used to treat coronary artery disease—coronary artery bypass graft (CABG) and percutaneous transluminal coronary angioplasty (PTCA)—were performed for elderly blacks at less than half the rate for whites. Two common orthopedic procedures—knee replacement and hip replacement—were also performed at a substantially lower rate for blacks.

Thromboendarterectomy is also shown in Table 4.5. This procedure, undertaken to treat occlusion of the carotid artery, was performed at a rate that was 67 percent lower for blacks than for whites. Disparities in thromboendarterectomy and sonography of the carotid artery—vis-a-vis the higher rate of stroke among blacks—raise concerns about the accessibility of referral-sensitive services for black beneficiaries who are at high risk of stroke.

Selected Eye Procedures

Elderly blacks have a lower rate than whites of cataract surgery, a common elective procedure to improve vision, but their rate of treatment of retinal lesions—a nonelective procedure to prevent sequelae that can lead to blindness—is much higher than whites (see Table 4.6, page 32). These findings are consistent with the information in Table 4.1, which shows fewer visits among blacks to ophthalmogists, and suggest that elderly blacks have less access to eye care than whites.

Table 4.5
Rates of Selected Cardiovascular and Orthopedic Procedures for Medicare Enrollees Age Sixty-five and Over, by Race, 1996

	White (rate per 1,000)	Black (rate per 1,000)	Ratio (black:white)
Coronary artery bypass graft	7.17	3.12	0.44
Percutaneous transluminal coronary angioplasty	9.16	4.49	0.49
Thrombo-endarterectomy	3.93	1.29	0.33
Total knee replacement	6.10	3.76	0.62
Total hip replacement	4.13	2.03	0.49

Source: Part B Monitoring System (age-adjusted rates), data supplied by Paul Eggers, Health Care Financing Administration.

TABLE 4.6

RATES OF SELECTED EYE PROCEDURES FOR MEDICARE ENROLLEES AGE SIXTY-FIVE AND OVER, BY RACE, 1996

	White (rate per 1,000)	Black (rate per 1,000)	Ratio (black:white)
Cataract removal/ lens insertion	57	42	0.72
Treatment of retinal lesions	10	16	1.56

Source: Part B Monitoring System (age-adjusted rates), data supplied by Paul Eggers, Health Care Financing Administration.

NONELECTIVE PROCEDURES ASSOCIATED WITH POOR OUTCOMES OF CHRONIC DISEASE

The three procedures shown in Table 4.7 are generally considered nonelective. Each is performed far more frequently for blacks than for whites. In 1994, for example, amputations of part or all of the lower limb were 3.47 times as frequent for blacks compared to whites. These differences reflect, in part, the fact that diabetes (an underlying factor) is 1.7 times as prevalent in elderly blacks as in whites. Yet the magnitude of the procedure rate for blacks compared to whites suggests that other factors are involved in the racial disparity in amputation rates.[6]

Arteriovenostomy procedures (shunts or cannulae implanted for renal dialysis) were 4.53 times as frequent for black beneficiaries as white beneficiaries, reflecting the greater prevalence of end-stage renal disease among blacks. The third procedure shown, excisional debridement, was performed 2.51 times as frequently for blacks as for whites. This procedure is performed for infection and skin breakdown, which are often adverse outcomes associated with quality of care.

The disparities in the rates for these three procedures are indications that elderly blacks are more likely to undergo procedures that reflect delayed diagnosis or treatment, less than optimal medical care, or failures in the management of chronic diseases.

Differences in Utilization by Socioeconomic Status

The effects of income on the use of elective services is often striking (see Table 4.8, page 34). In 1993, the ambulatory physician-visit rate among the least-affluent elderly whites (7.3 visits) was 19 percent lower than the rate for the most affluent whites (9.0 visits). But the least-well-off whites received 35 percent more emergency room visits than those best-off (data not shown).

The rates of use of Magnetic Resonance Imaging (MRI) and mammography among the least-affluent whites were 38 percent lower and 33 percent lower, respectively, than among the most affluent whites. Similarly, for blacks the differences were 27 percent lower for MRIs and 22 percent lower for mammography.

Among white and black beneficiaries, the rate of lower limb amputations rises as income declines. Among the least-affluent whites, this procedure was 47 percent more frequent than among the most affluent whites; among the least-affluent blacks, the rate of amputation was 21 percent greater than in the most affluent group.

Table 4.7
Three Procedures More Frequent among Black Medicare Beneficiaries than White Beneficiaries Age Sixty-five and Older, 1994

	White (rate per 1,000)	Black (rate per 1,000)	Ratio (black:white)
Amputation: lower limb	1.77	6.10	3.45
Arteriovenostomy	0.47	2.12	4.53
Excisional debridement	2.75	6.89	2.51

Source: Part A Monitoring System, data supplied by Paul Eggers, Health Care Financing Administration.

As noted, income distributions are substantially different between elderly blacks and elderly whites. When income distributions are standardized, differences between blacks and whites in Medicare utilization rates often diminish, although they do not entirely disappear.

TABLE 4.8
RATES FOR SELECTED SERVICES FOR MEDICARE BENEFICIARIES AGE SIXTY-FIVE AND OLDER, BY RACE AND INCOME, 1993

	AMBULATORY VISITS[a]	MRI[b]	MAMMOGRAPHY[b]	LOWER LIMB AMPUTATION[c]
White beneficiaries				
Total[d]	8.1	4.3	26.0	1.9
$20,501 and over	9.0	5.5	31.0	1.5
$16,301 to $20,500	8.3	4.4	27.2	1.8
$13,101 to $16,300	7.6	3.8	24.1	2.1
less than $13,001	7.3	3.4	20.8	2.2
Black beneficiaries				
Total[d]	7.2	3.5	17.1	6.7
$20,501 and over	8.0	4.5	20.4	5.8
$16,301 to $20,500	7.4	4.3	19.9	5.9
$13,101 to $16,300	7.7	4.3	21.1	6.1
less than $13,001	7.1	3.3	16.0	7.0
Ratio (black:white)				
Total	0.89	0.81	0.66	3.64
Income Adjusted	0.93	0.95	0.75	3.30

[a]rates per person
[b]rates per 100 persons; MRI = magnetic resonance imaging
[c]rates per 1,000 persons
[d]total rates adjusted for age

Source: *Monitoring the Impact of Medicare Physician Payment Reform on Utilization and Access; 1995 Report to Congress,* HCFA pub. no. 03379 (Baltimore, Md.: Health Care Financing Administration, 1995). For amputations, see Marian E. Gornick, et al., "Effects of Race and Income on Mortality and Use of Services among Medicare Beneficiaries," *New England Journal of Medicine* 335 (September 12, 1996): 791–99.

In summary, elderly blacks and the least affluent of both races have:

- lower rates of use of preventive services (for example, influenza immunizations) and health promotion services (for example, physicians' office visits);

- lower rates of use of certain tests (for example, colonoscopies) and elective surgeries (for example, coronary artery and major joint procedures); and

- higher rates of use of certain nonelective procedures that are associated with poor outcomes in the management of chronic conditions (for example, lower limb amputation).

5

What Are Probable Explanations for Disparities in Use?

Theories explaining disparities in economic and social variables—such as income, wealth, education, occupation, and health—generally center around the characteristics of different groups in the society and around the characteristics of the institutions of that society. In this chapter, before discussing the characteristics of the beneficiaries and the health care system that seem to be the most plausible explanations for disparities in Medicare use, certain factors are reviewed that ordinarily might be assumed to explain most of the disparities, but likely are not as important as other factors.

The type of health care delivery system is not likely to be a critical factor in explaining disparities in health care. In comparison to fee-for-service, HMOs and other managed care plans may be better organized to promote the overall use of preventive services, especially if HMOs are monitored by a reporting system that includes rates of preventive services. However, there is little information about the use of services in HMOs by race and socioeconomic status to compare with patterns found in the fee-for-service sector. One available study examined this issue by analyzing utilization in different types of health care plans and reported significant disparities in the use of cardiovascular procedures by blacks and Latinos in HMOs,[1] evidence that disparities occur in managed care as well.

In addition, there is not likely to be a particular feature of the Medicare program that explains a significant portion of the disparities in the use of service. Studies of the Veterans Administration (VA) programs also have found inequalities in the use of covered services. For example, VA studies have reported that procedures used to treat cardiovascular and cerebrovascular disease in VA hospitals were performed more frequently for white veterans than for black veterans.[2] Studies analyzing other health care programs have also shown variations in health care utilization across different subgroups.[3]

Similarly, financial barriers to care very likely cannot explain a significant portion of disparities in the use of Medicare services. Differences in mammogram use—which requires a 20 percent coinsurance payment—have been found to reflect, in part, differences by race and income in supplemental insurance.[4] However, the Medicare Current Beneficiary Survey (MCBS), which gathers information on sociodemographic and economic factors as well as insurance coverage, shows that mammography rates rise as income and education rise—even among those with supplemental insurance coverage.[5] Moreover, the MCBS shows that influenza immunization rates rise as income rises for this service—even though it requires no coinsurance.[6] The fact that minority beneficiaries and the least affluent of both races have lower rates of influenza immunization and mammography, even among those with additional insurance coverage, provides strong evidence that financial barriers are not the most important influences on disparities in the use of Medicare services by the elderly. Medicare findings are supported by a VA study showing that financial barriers cannot explain disparities in the use of certain procedures among veterans served in VA hospitals.[7]

It is also important to recognize that only a small fraction of disparities in health or health care can be explained by biological and clinical factors. For example, a study of six major risk factors—smoking, systolic blood pressure, cholesterol level, body-mass index, alcohol intake, and diabetes—showed that although blacks and whites differ in the prevalence of some risk factors, these six factors together could account for only 31 percent of the excess mortality between black and white adults, while income differences explained another 38 percent. The remaining 31 percent of the excess mortality remains unexplained.[8] One VA study showed that although blacks and whites differ in certain clinical factors, after adjusting for these differences black veterans were still 64 percent less likely than white veterans to undergo coronary artery bypass graft or percutaneous transluminal coronary angioplasty.[9] A Medicare study showed that although elderly blacks and whites differ in the prevalence of diabetes—a condition often underlying lower limb amputations—after accounting for difference in the rate of diabetes blacks still had a markedly higher rate of lower limb amputations than whites.[10]

Finally, racial and minority discrimination does not fully account for disparities in the use of Medicare services. Three facts support this statement. First, although disparities by race can be seen in the use of many elective services, the hospital admission rate for elderly blacks has increased faster than for whites. By 1986, the rate for blacks exceeded the rate for whites,[11] and by 1995 the rate for blacks was 15 percent higher than for whites, an indication that race alone cannot explain disparities in Medicare utilization. Second, racial disparities in the use of some services—such as mammography—decline when utilization rates are standardized by income, which means that socioeconomic differences play a role in explaining some of the racial disparities in Medicare use. Third, among elderly whites themselves there are disparities in the use of certain Medicare services. Rates of MRI and mammography decline as income declines, while lower limb amputations rise as income declines. Thus, Medicare analyses indicate that there is an association between several socioeconomic variables (including income, education, and supplemental insurance) and the use of Medicare services.[12] These factors, along with other cultural, social, and health system variables that are likely to play a role (discussed below), make it reasonable to believe that a multitude of factors—over and beyond the potential effects of race and minority discrimination—

influence Medicare utilization patterns. Although studies are available to shed some light on the influence of the factors discussed above, there are scarcely any studies to draw upon to identify—with any certainty—the factors that explain the major causes for disparities in Medicare utilization. However, the most plausible explanations, and the ones that best fit Medicare utilization patterns, are sociological. It must be underscored that the discussion that follows is based on theory and conjecture. Ultimately, data will be needed to test these potential explanations.

Beneficiary Characteristics That May Explain Some Disparities in Health Care Use

Beneficiary traits and cultural propensities—such as patient attitudes, beliefs, behaviors, and preferences—can be expected to range widely across the population aged sixty-five and over. At one end of the range are individuals with characteristics that are associated with a "culture of poverty"; at the other end are individuals with characteristics that are associated with what might be described as a "culture of advantage." A particular individual, of course, may exhibit traits associated with both cultures.

Certain characteristics prevailing among elderly persons living primarily in a culture of poverty may discourage them from initiating appointments with physicians to discuss a current health problem or to obtain a preventive service. For the elderly who live in poverty, a visit to a health care provider may require overcoming substantial obstacles posed by transportation and language difficulties. These obstacles may assume greater weight if the services are dispensed in an unsafe environment or in an environment lacking basic amenities.[13]

The culture of poverty, moreover, is generally associated with individuals who have acquired the least amount of knowledge about the value of preventive services and about specific symptoms of disease—such as indications of myocardial infarction or cancer—that warrant making an appointment to see a physician.[14] The lower use of health promotion services among the disadvantaged may also reflect certain attitudes, beliefs, and preferences. There is anecdotal evidence that the poor are more leery of the use of vaccines. Disadvantaged persons may also be more likely to see pain as part of the human condition, to be fatalistic about illness, and to assume that not much can be done to alter the course of disease. It may also be true that the poor tend to see medical care not as a necessity but as one of the luxuries of life. Thus, explanations about the lower use of health promotion services that are self-initiated, such as physicians' office visits, influenza immunizations, and mammograms are likely to involve, at least in part, the culture of poverty. Moreover, the culture of poverty may contribute to poorer health outcomes in the management of chronic conditions if the patient is not educated about the nature of the illness and the reasons for adherence to dietary and other management requirements.

Living in a culture of poverty can help to explain the less frequent use of self-initiated services and poorer outcomes of chronic conditions. But the theory of the culture of poverty cannot explain the consistent disparities found in the use of certain diagnostic and surgical procedures—such as colonoscopy, MRI, sonography of the carotid artery, coronary artery bypass graft, carotid endarterectomy, and hip and knee replacement—that can be recommended or referred and authorized only by physicians. These disparities in health care may be explained more satisfactorily by other hypotheses, including the complementary theory of the "culture of advantage." Just as socially advantaged individuals expect high-quality educational opportunities for their children and other societal opportunities, they also expect to receive high-quality medical care services. Living in a culture of advantage influences individuals to seek information about the latest available services and to expect consideration, fair treatment, and partnership with the established institutions in society, including the health care system. Accounts of the experience of advantaged individuals as they work their way through the maze of the health care system show how effective networks of friends and professionals can be in obtaining information about the best practitioners and institutions, and the latest diagnostic tests and procedures—

especially in times of serious illness.[15] These accounts often illustrate the beneficial effects of taking an active "ombudsman" role in health care, including making demands when services fall short of reasonable expectations. That affluent and educated individuals are able to obtain the latest and best health care available and have better health outcomes is consistent with the resources, privileges, opportunities, state of mind, and prestige that advantaged individuals command in every society. Moreover, as discussed next, the advantages that affluent and educated individuals have in obtaining high-quality health care are reinforced by certain characteristics of the health care delivery system.

Characteristics of the Health System That May Explain Some Disparities in Health Care

No substantial body of knowledge is available to identify the factors in our health care system that are directly associated with differences in the provision of health care services. The enormous complexities of the U.S. health care system make it difficult to untangle the factors in the system that influence the provision of services. However, physicians are among the most influential providers of health care. In the past, medical students have been drawn primarily from the upper and middle classes, and the majority have been white and male. Recently, there have been some shifts in the demographic composition of incoming classes of medical students (especially the increase in the number of females), and study is needed to understand these trends. Medical students choose the profession for reasons that include their interest in the science of medicine and their desire to help cure the illnesses of sick patients. Their academic training is concentrated in the biological sciences, with a relatively small focus on the social sciences. Their clinical training is concentrated on patients and the diagnosis and treatment of disease. The prestige afforded by the profession is likely to be attractive, particularly for those wishing to specialize, and students look forward to the rewarding life the profession brings.

Once in practice, physicians and allied health care providers develop formal and informal networks of colleagues, friends, and patients that contribute to a comfortable and profitable practice. Prestige and a stream of congenial referrals are more likely to come from advantaged patients than from poor, minority patients. In essence, physicians are likely to find interactions more comfortable and rewarding with patients who are advantaged like themselves than with disadvantaged patients. This is likely to have an impact on the effectiveness of patient care.

Sociologists have pointed out that our major institutions have not been successful in changing their ways in order to serve lower-class populations as effectively and constructively as more advantaged populations are served.[16] Because of this failure, culturally disadvantaged people may feel demeaned by various institutional practices such as waiting for long periods of time to see a physician and being given little explanation of their health problems and treatments.

In addition, the course of treatment physicians and other practitioners recommend to their patients may be influenced by stereotypical beliefs about the behavior of their patients. Physicians and other providers may believe that poor and minority patients are more likely to break appointments and to misunderstand complex information, and less likely to adhere to their orders. These perceptions may affect—perhaps subconsciously—the decision-making process and lead physicians to refrain from orders that require patient compliance and to hesitate before recommending certain procedures if they assume the patient does not live in an environment that is conducive to the aftercare needed for the best outcomes of the procedure. If highly technical and advanced services can be obtained only at a distant site, physicians may not hesitate to refer more advantaged patients to these sites but look for close-by alternatives if they assume that disadvantaged patients will not have the resources to travel to the site.

Whether minority or socioeconomic status of patients influences physicians in their recommendations and course of treatment is a question not often examined.[17] When physicians are evaluated, it is generally from the perspective of the outcomes of the care they provide individual patients. Hospitals, HMOs, and third-party payers may use different criteria in evaluating a physician's performance, but the focus is generally on the appropriateness and quality of the care provided to individual patients, not on the care provided to the population at risk. This approach leaves physicians and institutions largely unaware of the dramatic differences across population subgroups in the use of elective procedures, or in the use of nonelective procedures that are associated with poor outcomes of chronic conditions.

To keep abreast of the latest medical knowledge and to advance their skills, physicians look to their medical journals. The major medical journals concentrate on providing the latest scientific studies in the treatment of disease. Two widely circulated and prestigious journals—*The New England Journal of Medicine* and the *Journal of the American Medical Association*—cover a broad spectrum of medical issues and include articles that have a population-based focus, but they most frequently publish papers on the outcomes of treatment. Journals from the various specialty societies concentrate even more exclusively on clinical studies about the effectiveness of treatments. Publications that focus on health care delivery and health policy issues are not the journals practicing physicians follow; readership of health policy journals consists primarily of health services researchers and providers and others interested in public health and related areas. The average practicing physician is therefore likely to assume that the primary barrier to care is the lack of health insurance. Even health policy experts tend to discuss access to care in the United States in terms of the numbers of uninsured, to the neglect of the issue of disparities in health care among many of the insured.[18]

These conjectures about the underlying causes and explanations for disparities in Medicare utilization suggest that new initiatives, new approaches, and considerable new research are needed to bring about change. The final chapter discusses three recommendations that could begin to lessen the glaring disparities in Medicare utilization patterns.

6

What Steps Can Be Taken toward Bringing About a Change?

Medicare's continuing impact on the health and economic well-being of the elderly is widely acknowledged. It is clear, however, that the most vulnerable of the elderly are receiving less health care than they need to prevent illness and maintain health. Death rates for the three leading causes of death for persons sixty-five years of age and over—heart disease, cancer, and stroke—are greater for black beneficiaries than for white beneficiaries. No one knows with certainty how great a role health care might play in preventing the excess mortality blacks experience from these three causes of death. But Medicare data show conclusively that white beneficiaries receive more Medicare preventive services, tests, and elective procedures used to diagnose and treat these causes than black beneficiaries receive. The basic purpose of this paper in highlighting disparities in Medicare utilization and relating them to health outcomes is to arouse the interest of policy experts and the public to find ways to effect a change.

If we believe that individuals in the highest socioeconomic levels of society have the greatest advantage in obtaining optimal health care services, is there hope for improving access and equity in health care? The Medicare experience can speak to that issue. The conditions for participation in Medicare include the requirement that hospitals be in compliance with the Civil Rights Act of 1964, a condition that resulted in a rapid desegregation of hospitals when Medicare began. In the years preceding Medicare, half of the elderly were uninsured for hospital services, and illness could result in impoverishment and be a demeaning experience for those who had to depend on charity care. With the enactment of Medicare, the financial security of the elderly was greatly increased and the amount of charity care was greatly reduced. Over time, gaps in hospital discharge rates narrowed across subgroups of the elderly. Given the Medicare experience in influencing dramatic, long-lasting improvements in access to health care, we can expect further achievements. In essence, Medicare is a necessary condition for providing access to care, but Medicare alone is not sufficient. More needs to be done to ensure appropriate and effective use of services by all of the elderly needing care.

Although disparities in Medicare utilization have been the focus of several federal government reports as well as articles in the scientific literature, some cited in Chapter 4, these findings have not been widely disseminated to health policy experts, the health care community, or the public. The lack of awareness of these findings very likely contributes to the fact that disparities in Medicare utilization patterns have not changed much over time. As shown earlier, when Medicare began to cover influenza immunizations in 1993, only 17 percent of elderly blacks received flu shots, compared to 37 percent of whites—a black to white ratio of 0.47. In 1997, 24 percent of elderly blacks received flu shots, compared to 46 percent of whites—a black to white ratio of only 0.53. The record also shows that blacks continue to have lower rates of the common elective surgeries generally associated with improving health, and they continue to have substantially higher rates of certain nonelective procedures generally associated with poor management of chronic diseases.[1]

To take another giant step forward we need to make a start on accomplishing three goals.

Goal 1: Wide dissemination of information about patterns in Medicare use

We need to ensure that the public and the institutions that influence the delivery of health care acquire a body of knowledge about patterns of Medicare utilization and the most probable explanations for these patterns of use. It is important to accomplish this goal now because inequalities in utilization may increase with the growth of market-based systems oriented toward efficiency and profitability.

A broad-based strategy is needed to disseminate this information. To capture the attention of health policy experts, policymakers, and the public, we need a "white paper" from a respected institution—such as the Institute of Medicine—to begin a national discussion about disparities in health and health care and to call for policy changes. The call for change in the "white paper" needs to be followed up by reliable and widespread reports in newspapers, in magazines, on television, on the radio, on the Internet, and in publications for the elderly. These reports will attract public interest, especially among advocacy groups, and possibly inspire a national demand for new policies toward physician education and in the health care delivery system.

Goal 2: Development of data systems capable of monitoring equity in health care

We need to publicize the importance of establishing reliable and valid data systems for managed care. When the Medicare program began, it was structured around a uniform set of benefits, uniform payment methods, and health care delivered in the fee-for-service arena. This structure made it efficient to develop a data system from claims submitted for payment. During the twenty-five years that Medicare operated primarily as a fee-for-service program, this system was effective. With a growing percentage of the elderly (about 16 percent in 1998) enrolled in managed care plans, new data systems are needed.

Current approaches involving "report cards" that monitor overall rates of use of certain services are useful, but not sufficient. Many different types of services must be monitored—by socioeconomic status and racial/ethnic subgroups—in the managed care setting, or inequalities may go unrecognized.

Because claims are not a part of a managed care system, a major puzzle involves how to move away from the old method of generating information based on claims to a new method of generating information based on the managed care experience. Methods must also be devised to capture enrollee information not only on age, sex, and race, but on socioeconomic status as well.

Goal 3: Development of a Major Research and Experimentation Agenda

We need to develop a broad research agenda to expand knowledge about the specific characteristics of the beneficiaries and of the health care system that are associated with disparities in health care. Research and experimentation projects should focus on providing a better understanding of the pathways that lead to disparities in health care. A multitude of questions needs to be answered, such as to what extent are the recommendations made by health care providers associated with the race and socioeconomic status of the patients or with the race and socioeconomic status of the providers themselves? The health services research literature contains studies that can help guide new research toward identifying factors that underlie unequal use of health care services; for example, Hispanic women—whose rate of mammography in 1988 was only half the rate of white and black women—have reported far fewer physician recommendations for this procedure than other women.[2]

Education is likely to play a key role in diminishing disparities in health care. We need research relating to methods for outreach and education—especially in the use of preventive services such as influenza immunizations, as well as in the management of chronic diseases such as diabetes—and we need to test different approaches to identify ways of improving the use of Medicare services by vulnerable subgroups of the elderly.

We should begin now to put three or four initiatives and experiments in place. One such initiative is for the entire nation to be engaged in a campaign to eliminate disparities in influenza immunizations and mammography—including the community (for example, schools, churches, senior centers); the health care system (including physicians, hospitals, nurses, journals); the media (such as television, radio, newspapers); and families and friends (including spouses, children, neighbors)—in an all-out campaign.

Patterns of Medicare utilization are clear: The elderly most at risk of poor health—minorities and socially disadvantaged persons—receive fewer preventive services, fewer health promotion services, fewer tests to diagnose illness, and fewer surgeries that improve health and functioning. And, they undergo more last-resort procedures that are associated with poor outcomes of chronic disease. These patterns imply that although Medicare is a necessary condition for providing access to health care, it alone is not sufficient to ensure appropriate and effective use of covered services. Information about these Medicare utilization patterns has been available for nearly a decade, and it is time to take the necessary steps to bring about change.

NOTES

CHAPTER 1

1. The findings of three major studies that assess the early accomplishments of the Medicare program are summarized in Chapter 2.

2. The Medicare program maintains an ongoing data system for administrative purposes and for program evaluation. Known as the "administrative data," this data system contains information about the enrollees (for example, dates of entitlement, age, sex, race, and residence) and about services paid for by Medicare (information taken from the claims submitted for payment). Specific information about the health of the enrollee is not generally available from the administrative data, nor is utilization information available for beneficiaries enrolled in HMOs. To obtain additional information for program administration and evaluation, the Medicare program sponsors an ongoing survey—known as the Medicare Current Beneficiary Survey (MCBS)—to collect socioeconomic and health information for a sample of beneficiaries.

3. The terms "hospital discharge rate" and "hospital admission rate" are often used interchangeably to mean the number of hospitalizations per 1,000 persons per year. In compiling Medicare statistics, the hospital discharge rate is generally used and it refers to the number of discharges between January 1 and December 31 in a specific year per 1,000 enrollees.

4. Lu Ann Aday, Gretchen Fleming, and Ronald Andersen, *Access to Medical Care in the U.S.; Who Has It, Who Doesn't?* (Chicago: Pluribus Press, Inc., and the University of Chicago, Center for Health Administration Studies, 1984).

5. Health information is available from various federal agencies, including the National Cancer Institute and the National Center for Health Statistics, that generate nationwide data on different measures of health (alternatively called "health status" or "health outcomes")—such as mortality and morbidity rates—by age, sex, race, and other characteristics.

The primary source of Medicare utilization information is the Medicare administrative data system, which became operational with the implementation of Medicare in 1966. Certain components of the administrative data are the foundation for their strength and usefulness. A major component of the administrative data is the enrollment file, containing information on every person ever enrolled in the program, including date and type of entitlement and date of death (if applicable). Separate claims files are maintained containing information on the use of Medicare-covered services. The utilization data are extracted from claims submitted for payment; this information can be linked by a unique identifier to information in the enrollment files. When Medicare began, all of the enrollees received services on a fee-for-service basis, and the Medicare administrative data represented the use and costs of covered services for all of the elderly in the nation.

Although enrollment information continues to be maintained for all Medicare enrollees, utilization information on a service by service basis has not been available for HMO enrollees because payment to HMOs is on a capitated basis. Enrollment in HMOs has been growing, reaching about 16 percent of the total elderly enrolled in Medicare in January 1998. If HMO enrollment continues to grow, Medicare's administrative data will reflect the utilization experience for a decreasing percentage of enrollees.

Despite this and other limitations, the Medicare administrative data have been an invaluable source of information on the use and costs of Medicare services since the program began. The data system is a primary source of information for program administration and evaluation, including program statistics, trend analyses, actuarial projections, and the establishment of payment formulas. Its data may be used to conduct a wide array of studies and demonstrations.

6. Currently, very little data is available to compare utilization patterns in HMOs with fee-for-service patterns.

CHAPTER 2

1. Paul Starr, *The Social Transformation of American Medicine* (New York: Basic Books, 1982), pp. 261, 373.

2. Herman M. Somers and Anne R. Somers, *Medicare and the Hospitals* (Washington, D.C.: The Brookings Institution, 1967), p. 4.

3. Starr, *The Social Transformation of American Medicine,* p. 373.

4. Ibid.

5. See Chapter 1, note 2.

6. Regina Loewenstein, "Early Effects of Medicare on the Health Care of the Aged," *Social Security Bulletin* (April 1971): 3–21.

7. Stephen H. Long and Russell F. Settle, "Medicare and the Disadvantaged Elderly: Objectives and Outcomes," *Milbank Memorial Fund Quarterly/Health and Society* 62, no. 4 (1984): 609–56. These authors hypothesized that racial differences in the pre-Medicare period might reflect the greater proportion of nonwhites living in rural and inner-city areas, which had relatively fewer medical resources, and in the segregated South. (After Title VI of the 1964 Civil Rights Act, segregated institutions were no longer able to receive federal funds. Because participation in Medicare required provider compliance with Title VI and the vast majority of hospitals applied to participate, almost overnight Medicare brought an end to segregation in hospitals.)

8. Martin Ruther and Allen Dobson, "Equal Treatment and Unequal Benefits: A Re-Examination of the Use of Medicare Services by Race, 1967–1976," *Health Care Financing Review* 2, no. 3 (1981): 55–83.

9. Ruther and Dobson, "Equal Treatment and Unequal Benefits," reported one finding (p. 61) whose significance was largely overlooked: that nonwhite beneficiaries had substantially fewer services by orthopedic surgeons, radiologists, and internists. In hindsight this finding was a first indication that treatment patterns differed across subgroups of the elderly.

10. Avedis Donabedian, "Effects of Medicare and Medicaid on Access to and Quality of Health Care," *Public Health Reports* 91, no. 4 (July–August 1976): 322–31.

11. Karen Davis, "Inequality and Access to Health Care," *The Milbank Quarterly* 69, no. 69 (1991): 253–73.

12. A. Marshall McBean and Marian Gornick, "Differences by Race in the Rates of Procedures Performed in Hospitals for Medicare Beneficiaries," *Health Care Financing Review* 15, no. 4 (1994): 77–90.

CHAPTER 3

1. For a broad overview of the associations between socioeconomic status and health, see John P. Bunker, Deanna S. Gomby, and Barbara H. Kehrer, eds., *Pathways to Health: The Role of Social Factors,* a conference sponsored by the Henry J. Kaiser Family Foundation, Menlo Park, Calif., March 25–27, 1987.

2. E. Pamuk et al., "Socioeconomic Status and Health Chartbook," in *Health, United States, 1998* (Hyattsville, Md.: National Center for Health Statistics, 1998).

3. Ibid, p. 441. In 1976, all federal data systems began to use four racial groups and one ethnic category: American Indian or Alaskan Native; Asian or Pacific Islander; Black; White; and Hispanic origin, which includes persons of all races. In the early years of the Medicare program, three categories were used to classify enrollees by race: white, black, and all other races. Efforts are being made to update Medicare administrative data to conform to the federal data system requirements.

4. Kyriakos S. Markides, "Mortality and Morbidity Among Hispanic Elderly." (Paper presented at the Workshop on Racial and Ethnic Differences in Health in Late Life in the United States, Washington, D.C., December 12–13, 1994).

5. Mortality rates are generally considered the most reliable measures of health, but they are subject to misreporting and other errors. They are derived from deaths reported by states (used as numerators) and from U.S. census data (used as denominators). Consistency between race identification on death certificates and census data is relatively high for whites and blacks, but inconsistencies are estimated to result in death rates that are about 12 percent too low for Asians and about 7 percent too low for Hispanics. Among older groups, age is often misreported as well. The leading causes of death provide insight into the effects of various conditions on subgroups of the population.

Illness or morbidity rates describe incidence or prevalence of a specific disease and are derived from various sources, including surveys, registries, and medical records. Differences in illness rates across subgroups can reflect access to care—that is, whether an individual has seen a physician and been diagnosed as well as informed and treated for a particular condition, such as diabetes, hypertension, or glaucoma.

Disability rates are used to compare health status across groups and are derived from a variety of sources. Measures often used for analyzing disability are "activities of daily living" (ADLs), which include activities such as the ability to bathe and walk, and "instrumental activities of daily living" (IADLs), which include activities such as the ability to perform household chores, use the telephone, and to shop.

Self-reported health status is frequently collected in household surveys. Self-reported health status (typically excellent, good, fair, poor) has been shown to correlate with mortality, morbidity, and disability rates for these groups. Some of the disparities in health across subgroups may reflect different tendencies among subgroups in the way they assess their health in relation to others.

6. Diane B. Dutton and Sol Levine, "Socioeconomic Status and Health: Overview, Methodological Critique and Reformation," in Bunker, Gomby, and Kehrer, *Pathways to Health*.

7. Markides, "Mortality and Morbidity Among Hispanic Elderly."

8. The focus in our society on the health of black Americans reflects the interest in our nation in alleviating the profound impacts of slavery. Similarly, interest in the health of American Indians reflects our interest in reversing the negative impacts from the settlement of America. These special concerns are reflected in the current effort by the U.S. Department of Health and Human Services to promote health through an initiative known as "Healthy People 2000." National goals have been established to increase the span of healthy life, reduce health disparities among Americans, and achieve access to preventive services for all Americans. The 1995–96 progress report described the gains made in eliminating racial and ethnic disparities for twenty-seven conditions.

9. See Laura E. Montgomery and Olivia Carter-Pokras, "Health Status by Social Class and/or Minority Status: Implications for Environmental Equity Research," *Toxicology and Industrial Health* 9, no. 5 (1993): 729–73.

Chapter 4

1. Health Care Financing Administration, *Health Care Financing: Special Report: Hospital Data by Geographic Area for Aged Medicare Beneficiaries: Selected Procedures, 1986,* vol. 2, HCFA publication no. 03301 (Washington, D.C.: Government Printing Office, 1990).

2. The classification system, which was devised by HCFA and the Urban Institute, is known as the Berenson-Eggers system. For a discussion of this system see Paul Eggers, "Beneficiary Access and Utilization," Appendix II, in *Monitoring the Impact of Medicare Physician Payment Reform on Utilization and Access; 1994 Report to Congress,* HCFA publication no. 03358 (Baltimore: Health Care Financing Administration, 1994).

3. See Jonathan C. Javitt et al., "Undertreatment of Glaucoma among Black Americans," *New England Journal of Medicine* 325 (November 14, 1991): 1418–22.

4. See A. Marshall McBean, John D. Babish, and Joan L. Warren, "The Impact and Cost of Influenza in the Elderly," *Archives of Internal Medicine* 153 (September 27, 1993): 2105–11.

5. See Marian E. Gornick et al., "Effects of Race and Income on Mortality and Use of Services among Medicare Beneficiaries," *New England Journal of Medicine* 335 (September 12, 1996): 791–99.

6. For a fuller discussion of racial and income disparities in the use of Medicare services, see Gornick et al., "Effects of Race and Income on Mortality and Use of Services Among Medicare Beneficiaries." See also A. Marshall McBean and Marian Gornick, "Differences by Race in the Rates of Procedures Performed in Hospitals for Medicare Beneficiaries," *Health Care Financing Review* 15, no. 4 (1994): 77–90.

Chapter 5

1. David M. Carlisle, Barbara D. Leake, and Martin F. Shapiro, "Racial and Ethnic Disparities in the Use of Cardiovascular Procedures: Associations with Types of Health Insurance," *American Journal of Public Health* 87, no. 2 (February 1997): 263–67.

2. Jeff Whittle et al., "Racial Differences in the Use of Invasive Cardiovascular Procedures in the Department of Veterans Affairs Medical System," *New England Journal of Medicine* 329 (August 26, 1993): 621–27; Eric D. Peterson et al., "Racial Variation in Cardiac Procedure Use and Survival Following Acute Myocardial Infarction in the Department of Veterans Affairs," *Journal of the American Medical Association* 271 (April 20, 1994): 1175–80.

3. Mark B. Wenneker and Arnold M. Epstein, "Racial Inequalities in the Use of Procedures for Patients with Ischemic Heart Disease in Massachusetts," *Journal of the American Medical Association* 261, no. 2 (January 13, 1989): 253–57. See also Noralou P. Roos and Cameron A. Mustard, "Variations in Health and Health Care Use by Socioeconomic Status in Winnipeg, Canada: Does the System Work Well? Yes and No," *Milbank Quarterly* 75, no. 1 (1997): 89–111; and Ronnie D. Horner, Eugene Z. Oddone, and David B. Matchar, "Theories Explaining Racial Differences in the Utilization of Diagnostic and Therapeutic Procedures for Cerebrovascular Disease," *Milbank Quarterly* 73, no. 3 (1995): 443–62.

4. Jan Blustein, "Medicare Coverage, Supplemental Insurance, and the Use of Mammography by Older Women," *New England Journal of Medicine* 332 (April 27, 1995): 1138–43.

5. Ibid.

6. Marian E. Gornick et al., "Effects of Race and Income on Mortality and Use of Services among Medicare Beneficiaries," *New England Journal of Medicine* 335 (September 12, 1996): 791–99.

7. Whittle et al., "Racial Differences in the Use of Invasive Cardiovascular Procedures in the Department of Veterans Affairs Medical System."

8. Mac W. Otten, Jr. et al., "The Effect of Known Risk Factors on the Excess Mortality of Black Adults in the U.S.," *Journal of the American Medical Association* 263 (February 9, 1990): 845–50. Some writers on this issue believe that income inequalities are the major risk-factor for inequalities in health outcomes. See Richard G. Wilkinson, *Unhealthy Societies: The Afflictions of Inequalities* (London: Routledge, 1996).

9. Peterson et al., "Racial Variation in Cardiac Procedure Use and Survival Following Acute Myocardial Infarction in the Department of Veterans Affairs."

10. Gornick et al., "Effects of Race and Income on Mortality and Use of Services among Medicare Beneficiaries." See also Edward Guadagnoli et al., "The Influence of Race on the Use of Surgical Procedures for Treatment of Peripheral Vascular Disease of the Lower Extremities," *Archives of Surgery* 130 (April 1995): 381–86.

11. Marshall McBean and Marian E. Gornick, "Differences by Race in the Rates of Procedures Performed in Hospitals for Medicare Beneficiaries," *Health Care Financing Review* 15, no. 4 (1994): 77–90.

12. The Medicare Current Beneficiary Survey (MCBS) is useful for multivariate analyses of services that have high rates of utilization such as overall hospital admission rates, flu immunizations, or mammography. However, the MCBS cannot be used for multivariate analyses of common surgeries, such as coronary artery bypass graft, because the number of these surgeries in the sample is too low. The size of the Medicare administrative data system makes it feasible to study the use of specific services across subgroups of the elderly. As shown in this chapter, by linking Medicare administrative data to aggregate data from the U.S. census on a ZIP code basis, the use of specific services was studied by income. However, collinearity between income and education in the aggregate census data ruled out studying the separate effects of income and education.

13. William C. Cockerham, *Medical Sociology* (Englewood Cliffs, N.J.: Prentice-Hall, 1978). See especially Chapter 4, "The Process of Seeking Care."

14. See Chapter 2, "Patterns of Access to Health Care," in *Securing Access to Health Care: President's Commission for the Study of Ethical Problems in Medicine and Biomedical and Behavioral Research, vol. 1: Report* (Washington, D.C.: U.S. Government Printing Office, 1983).

15. See, for example, Martha Weinman Lear, *Heartsounds* (New York: Simon and Schuster, 1980).

16. Lee Rainwater, "The Problem of Lower Class Culture," in Daniel P. Moynihan, ed., *On Understanding Poverty: Perspectives from the Social Sciences* (New York: Basic Books, 1969).

17. See Kevin A. Schulman et al., "The Effect of Race and Sex on Physicians' Recommendations for Cardiac Catheterization," *New England Journal of Medicine* 340 (February 25, 1999): 618–26.

18. Beginning January 7, 1999, *The New England Journal of Medicine* devoted a series of health policy articles to "The American Health Care System." It included a broad overview of issues in the current Medicare program, but did not discuss disparities in utilization.

Chapter 6

1. In 1986, for coronary artery bypass graft, the black to white ratio was 0.28. By 1992, the ratio increased to 0.39. In 1996, it was 0.43. For amputation of part or all of the lower limb, the black to white ratio in 1986 was 3.24, in 1992, 3.62, and in 1996, 3.47. (Source for 1986 and 1992: A. Marshall McBean and Marian Gornick, "Differences By Race in the Rates of Procedures Performed in Hospitals for Medicare Beneficiaries," *Health Care Financing Review* 15, no. 4 [1994]: 77–90; unpublished data from Health Care Financing Administration [1996] supplied by Paul Eggers.)

2. Sarah A. Fox and Judith A. Stein, "The Effect of Physician-Patient Communication on Mammography Utilization by Different Ethnic Groups," *Medical Care* 29, no. 11 (November 1991): 1065–81.

Index

Note: Page numbers followed by *t* and *n* refer to tables and notes respectively.

About the Author

Marian E. Gornick worked for over twenty years at the Health Care Financing Administration (HCFA), where she was responsible for the design and development of a research agenda to study public policy issues relating to the Medicare and Medicaid programs, especially the impact of these programs on the beneficiaries. Since leaving HCFA she has continued her analyses of disparities in the use of Medicare services at the Georgetown Public Policy Institute under a grant awarded by The Commonwealth Fund. She has published several studies and has written papers tracing the history and evaluating the impact of the Medicare program, including three studies analyzing the effects of Medicare on beneficiaries after ten years, twenty years, and thirty years of program operation; and in the past decade she has published reports about disparities in the use of Medicare services, one of which became the focus of an ABC evening news program.